Intermittent Fasting for Women Over 50

2021

A complete guide for women to reduce their health risks with intermittent fasting techniques and remain healthy after 50

LUNA THORNTON

© **Copyright 2021 LUNA THORNTON- All rights reserved.**

This document is geared towards providing exact and reliable information in regard to the topic and issue covered. The publication is sold with the idea that the publisher is not required to render accounting, officially permitted, or otherwise, qualified services. If advice is necessary, legal or professional, a practiced individual in the profession should be ordered.

From a Declaration of Principles which was accepted and approved equally by a Committee of the American Bar Association and a Committee of Publishers and Associations.

In no way is it legal to reproduce, duplicate, or transmit any part of this document in either electronic means or in printed format. Recording of this publication is strictly prohibited, and any storage of this document is not allowed unless with written permission from the publisher. All rights reserved.

The information provided herein is stated to be truthful and consistent, in that any liability, in terms of inattention or otherwise, by any usage or abuse of any policies, processes, or directions contained within is the solitary and utter responsibility of the recipient reader. Under no circumstances

will any legal responsibility or blame be held against the publisher for any reparation, damages, or monetary loss due to the information herein, either directly or indirectly? Respective authors own all copyrights not held by the publisher.

The information herein is offered for informational purposes solely and is universal as such. The presentation of the information is without a contract or any type of guarantee assurance.

The trademarks that are used are without any consent, and the publication of the trademark is without permission or backing by the trademark owner. All trademarks and brands within this book are for clarifying purposes only and are owned by the owners themselves, not affiliated with this document.

Contents

Introduction 6

CHAPTER 1: What is Intermittent Fasting? 10

    1.1 Humans and fasting 10

    1.2 Fasting and Religion 13

    1.3 Fasting as a form of protest 15

    1.4 Popular Intermittent Fasting Methods 17

    1.5 Spontaneous meal skipping 29

    1.6 The effects of Intermittent Fasting on Cells and Hormones 30

    1.7 Intermittent fasting is a very powerful weight-loss tool .. 33

    1.8 Who should be careful or avoid it? 35

    1.9 Safety and Side Effects 35

    1.10 Some popular questions and answers on Intermittent Fasting 36

    1.11 Intermittent fasting coupled with excellent ways to help lose weight after 50 38

CHAPTER 2: Intermittent Fasting and its Health Benefits For Women Over 50 50

    2.1 Intermittent Fasting 52

    2.2 The Technique 54

    2.3 Best Intermittent Fasting Types for Women 57

    2.4 Getting started is quite easy 59

    2.5 Safety and Benefits of Intermittent Fasting 60

    2.6 How to succeed with an intermittent fasting protocol 68

CHAPTER 3: A Guide For Women Over 50 On How To Start 70

    3.1 Intermittent fasting may affect men and women differently 71

    3.2 Health benefits of intermittent fasting for women 72

3.3 How does intermittent fasting work? 75

3.4 What makes intermittent fasting work? 76

3.5 Is intermittent fasting healthy?..................................... 77

3.6 Is intermittent fasting the best technique? 78

3.7 You can lead a care-free life... 79

3.8 Tips to keep an intermittent fasting diet on track 79

3.9 The best foods to eat on an Intermittent Fasting diet 84

3.10 Best drinks for intermittent fasting 86

3.11 The drinks that you must avoid during intermittent fasting 97

3.12 Intermittent fasting side effects 104

3.13 Why does intermittent fasting result in constipation in some people? 106

3.14 What if you're having the problem of diarrhea?.......... 108

3.15 Keep your bowel movements regular while you are on intermittent fasting... 108

Conclusion 111

Introduction

Intermittent fasting is avidly practiced by women over 50 to overcome their age-related issues. It is also called intermittent energy restrictions. In intermittent fasting, you have the liberty to choose from various timing schedules of meals that cycle between voluntary fasting & non-fasting in a specific period. The popularity of the intermittent fasting technique for women over 50 years of age has grown tremendously in recent years. Intermittent fasting, in contrast to other diets, relies on when to eat by aligning daily short-term fasts into the routine. This eating style can assist you in consuming fewer calories, losing weight, and reducing your risk of diabetes and heart disease. Intermittent fasting (IF) is a form of eating that alternates between fasting and regular eating. Fasting on alternating days, regular 16-hour fasts, or fasting for twenty-four hours two days a week are the most common practices. Intermittent fasting, unlike most diets, does not require calorie or macronutrient monitoring. In fact, there are no dietary or dietary restrictions, making it more of a way of living than a diet. Intermittent fasting is a popular way to lose weight since it is an easy, quick, and inexpensive way to eat little but lose body fat. It may also aid in the prevention of heart disease and diabetes, the maintenance of muscle mass, and the enhancement of psychological well-being. Furthermore, since there are few meals to plan, prepare and serve, this eating style will help you save time in the kitchen. Intermittent fasting is a form of eating that involves periodic, short-term fasting. It's a common way of life that can help with weight loss, body composition, disease prevention, and overall well-being. Intermittent fasting will help you shed weight while still lowering the risk of contracting a host of chronic diseases. The main cause of death in the world is heart disease. It aids in the improvement of heart wellbeing. High blood pressure, high LDL cholesterol, and high triglyceride levels are three of the most common risk factors for cardiac failure. Intermittent fasting reduced blood pressure by 6 percent in just eight weeks in a sample of 16 obese men and women. Intermittent fasting also reduced LDL cholesterol by 25percent and triglycerides by 32%, according to the same report. Intermittent fasting will also help you treat your diabetes and lower your chances of contracting it. Intermittent fasting, including prolonged calorie restriction, tends to reduce some diabetes risk factors. It mostly accomplishes this by lowering insulin levels and decreasing insulin tolerance. When done correctly, intermittent fasting can be an easy and efficient way to lose weight since short-term fasts will help you consume few calories and lose weight. Several studies have found that intermittent fasting is just as effective as standard calorie-restricted diets for weight loss in the short term. Intermittent fasting resulted in an overall weight loss of fifteen pounds over a period of three to twelve months, according to a 2018 study of research in overweight adults. Over a span of 3–24 weeks, intermittent fasting decreased body weight by three to eight percent in overweight or obese individuals, according to another report. Switching to intermittent fasting may help you eat less naturally. Intermittent fasting has been shown in several trials to suppress essential markers of inflammation. Chronic inflammation can cause weight gain and a slew of other health issues. In one study, eight weeks of intermittent fasting reduced stress and binge eating habits in obese adults while enhancing body appearance. Intermittent fasting has been shown to extend lifespan by 33–83 percent in rats and mice. When compared to prolonged calorie restriction, intermittent fasting tends to be more efficient at maintaining muscle mass. And when you're at rest, having more muscle mass makes you eat more calories. Intermittent fasting can improve weight loss and lower the risk of heart disease and diabetes in women. Intermittent fasting (IF) is one of the most popular health and fitness trends in the world right now. It is being used by people to lose weight, improve their health, and simplify their lives. It has been shown in numerous studies to have powerful effects on the body and brain and may even help you live longer. This book contains valuable information for leading a healthy and satisfying life for women over 50.

CHAPTER 1: What is Intermittent Fasting?

Intermittent fasting (IF) is a type of eating that alternates between fasting and eating periods. It's very trendy in the fitness and health community right now. It doesn't tell you which foods to eat, but instead when you should eat them. In this sense, it's more adequately defined as an eating pattern rather than a diet in the traditional sense. Daily sixteen-hour fasts or fasting for 24 hours twice a week are two common intermittent fasting methods.

1.1 Humans and fasting

Fasting is defined as abstaining from drink or food, or even both, for the purposes of health, ritual, religion, or ethics. Abstinence can be total or partial, long or short, continuous or intermittent. Fasting is promoted & practiced by physicians, religious founders & followers, culturally chosen individuals (such as hunters or applicants for the initiation rites), & groups or individuals as a way of protesting against what they consider are breaches of social, political or ethical principles since antiquity. Fasting is used therapeutically ever since the 5th-century B.C.E, at least when Hippocrates, a Greek physician, advised abstinence from drink and food for patients with certain indications of the illness. Some doctors recognized fasting instinct, in which patients with certain diseases naturally lose their appetite. Fasting was believed to be an important natural part of the recovery process, so some doctors believed that giving food during such states was inappropriate and possibly even harmful. In the latter half of the nineteenth century, some of the 1st organized training of fasting in humans and animals began to emerge, and a better understanding of the physiological effects of fasting began to emerge. As more was learned about nutrition as well as nutritional necessities of the human body in the twentieth century, fasting methods became more sophisticated, & a diverse range of approaches arose. Fasting was, for example, used as treatment & a method to prevent disease in a variety of settings (in a clinic or home or hospital). Few fasting methods, especially those used to treat chronic diseases, which lasted for about a month, permitted only calories-free tea or water to be consumed & included exercise & enemas. Some Other methods, referred to as the modified fasting, that allowed for intake of 500 to 200 calories in a day (daily calories requirements of the adult's variety from about 3,000 to 1,600 calories, based on age, sex, as well as activity level). Moreover, fasting sometimes included spiritual or psychological therapy; depending upon the method used, the calories were usually in the form of vegetable broth, bread, fruit juice, and so on; depending on the method used, calories were usually in the form of, vegetable broth, bread fruit juice, and so altered fasting were differentiated from the very less-calorie diet, that permitted up to 800 kcal per day & was typically used to lose a lot of weight. Intermittent fasting usually consisted of cyclic times of the calorie restriction, like a 24-hour fast followed by a 24-hr period of normal calorie consumption. Although fasting was clearly applicable in few cases of the disease, like some acute diseases (especially when followed quickly by loss of appetite), and whether fasting was helpful to human health in other cases remained unclear by the twenty-first century. For example, while studies in humans showed that intermittent fasting for fifteen days enhanced insulin-mediated sugar uptake into the tissues, the studies in the rodents showed that long-term intermittent fasting encouraged glucose intolerance as well as the release of harmful oxidants from the tissues.

1.2 Fasting and Religion

Fasting was a practice in ancient peoples' & civilizations' religions to prepare people, particularly priestesses and priests, to approach gods. Gods were considered to unveil the divine teaching in the dreams & visions just after fast, which required total devotion from the devotees in Hellenistic mystery religions (– for example, the healing cult of the god Asclepius). Fasting was often one of the prerequisites for penance among Peru's pre-Columbian peoples after they confessed their sins to priest.

In most cultures, the practice was seen as a way to appease an enraged deity or even to help in the resurrecting of the deity who had died (for example, vegetation god). Fasting was performed during and before the vision quest in the religions of some Native American tribes. Shamans (religious figures believed to have the ability to heal & communicate psychically) among the Evenk of Siberia frequently received their first visions following an unexplained illness. They fasted & prepared themselves to understand even more visions and control spirits after the initial vision. Prior to major ceremonies associated with seasonal changes, priestly societies amongst all the Pueblo Indians of the American Southwest used to fast during retreats. Fasting for specific purposes or beforehand or during sacred periods has long been a feature of the world's major religions. Fasting with certain prescribed instructions and practicing specific types of meditation, for example, leads to the trances that allow people to detach themselves from the world & reach a transcendent state in Jainism. As a component of the meditation practices, some Theravada Buddhist monks fast. Sadhus (the holy men) in India are applauded for the frequent private fasts for a variety of reasons. Only Zoroastrianism restricts fasting among Western religions, believing that such asceticism won't aid faithful in the fight against evil. Fasting is emphasized in other Western faiths, including Christianity, Judaism, and Islam. Several annual fast days are observed by Judaism, which developed most dietary laws & customs, primarily on the days of the penitence (like Yom Kippur, Day of the Atonement) or grief. During Lent, spring periods of the penitence before Easter, & Advent, penitential periods before Christmas,

Christians, particularly Roman Catholics and Eastern Orthodox, observe a 40-day fast. Since the 2nd Vatican Council (in 1962–65), Roman Catholics' observance has been modified to allow more individual choices, with compulsory fasting just on Ash Wednesdays and Good Fridays during Lent. Individual members of the church are usually left to decide whether or not to fast in Protestant churches. In Islam, the month of Ramadhan is a time of penitence & complete fasting from morning to night.

1.3 Fasting as a form of protest

Fasting can be useful in describing social & political views, mainly as a sign of solidarity or protest, in addition to its religious role. Mahatma Gandhi set the standard for this approach when he fasted in prison in the early twentieth century to compensate for the violent excesses of his supporters who didn't follow the teachings of satyagraha (the nonviolence) in the face of British control in India. Later Gandhi fasted several times in pursuit of similar goals, including the removal of government-imposed restrictions on untouchables. So, Fasting has been used to protest war & what are perceived to be social evils & injustices, such as the fasts of black American comedian Dick Geregory in the 1960s in the protest of violations of American Indian civil rights and US military activities in Southeast Asia. During hunger strikes to demand acknowledgment of themselves along with the associates as the political prisoners, ten Irish nationalists died in a Belfast prison in 1981.

Bottom line

Fasting has been practiced by humans since the beginning of time. Supermarkets, refrigerators, and year-round food were not available to ancient hunter-gatherers. They couldn't always find something to eat. As a result, humans have evolved to be able to exist for long periods of time without food. Fasting is, in fact, more natural than eating three to four (or more) meals per day on a regular basis. Fasting is also practiced in Islam, Christianity, Judaism, and Buddhism for religious or spiritual reasons.

1.4 Popular Intermittent Fasting Methods

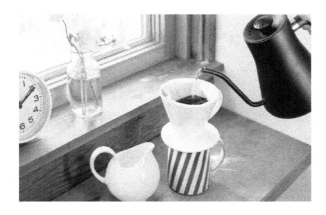

Consistent, short-term fasts and periods of minimal or no food consumption — are part of an eating pattern known as intermittent fasting. Intermittent fasting is commonly thought of as a weight-loss strategy. People who fast for short periods of time consume fewer calories, which may lead to weight loss over time. Intermittent fasting, on the other hand, may help reduce risk factors for diabetes and cardiovascular disease by decreasing cholesterol as well as blood sugar levels. Intermittent fasting can be done in a variety of ways. All of the methods entail dividing the day or week into periods of eating and fasting. You eat nothing or very little at all during the fasting periods. All methods can be successful, but determining which one works best for you is a personal decision. The most popular methods are listed below to assist you in selecting the method that best suits your lifestyle.

The 16/8 method

	DAY 1	DAY 2	DAY 3	DAY 4	DAY 5	DAY 6	DAY 7
Midnight							
4 AM	FAST	FAST	FAST	FAST	FAST	FAST	FAST
8 AM							
12 PM	First meal	First meal	First meal	First meal	First meal	First meal	First meal
4 PM	Last meal by 8pm	Last meal by 8pm	Last meal by 8pm	Last meal by 8pm	Last meal by 8pm	Last meal by 8pm	Last meal by 8pm
8 PM	FAST	FAST	FAST	FAST	FAST	FAST	FAST
Midnight							

THE 16/8 METHOD

Fitness expert Martin Berkhan popularized this method, which is also known as the Leangains protocol. It entails skipping breakfast and limiting your daily eating time to 8 hours, such as between 1 and 9 p.m. After that, you fast for 16 hours. You can eat two, three, or even four meals within the eating window. One of the most popular fasting plans for weight loss is the intermittent fasting 16/8 plan. Food & calorie-containing drinks are restricted to an 8-hour window per day under the plan. It necessitates fasting for the remaining 16 hrs. of the day. While the other diets may have strict rules & regulations, the 16/8 technique is more flexible and based on a time-limited feeding model. You can consume calories during any 8-hour period. Some people will avoid eating late and adhere to a 9 a.m. to 5 p.m. schedule, while others skip breakfast and fast from noon to 8 p.m. Limiting the number of hours you can consume during the day may aid in weight loss and blood pressure reduction. It's as simple as not eating anything else after dinner and skipping breakfast to follow this fasting method. If you eat the last meal at 8 p.m. and don't eat again till noon the next day, you'll have fasted for 16 hours. Women are generally advised to fast for only fourteen to fifteen hours since they seem to do very well with shorter fasts. This method may be difficult to adjust to at first for people who get hungry in the morning and want to eat breakfast. Many breakfast-skippers, on the other hand, eat in this manner instinctively. During the fast, you can drink coffee, water and other low-calorie beverages to help you feel less hungry. It's critical to focus on eating healthy foods during your eating window. If you eat a lot of junk food or consume an excessive number of calories, this method will not work. According to research, time-restricted feeding patterns, such as the 16/8 method, can help prevent hypertension and reduce food consumption, resulting in weight loss. The 16/8 method, when combined with resistance training, helped male participants lose fat and maintain muscle mass, according to a 2016 study. A more recent study discovered that the 16/8 method had no effect on muscle or strength gains in women doing resistance training. While the 16/8 method can be easily incorporated into any lifestyle, several other people may find it difficult to go 16 hours without eating. Furthermore, eating too many snacks as well as junk food during the 8-hour fasting window can counteract the benefits of 16/8 intermittent fasting. To reap the most health benefits from this diet, eat a well-balanced diet rich in fruits, whole grains, vegetables, healthy fats and protein. Almost all people have found the 16/8 method to be the most straightforward, long-term, and simple to follow. It's also the most well-known.

The 5:2 diet

THE 5:2 DIET							
DAY 1	DAY 2	DAY 3	DAY 4	DAY 5	DAY 6	DAY 7
Eats normally	Women: 500 calories Men: 600 calories	Eats normally	Eats normally	Women: 500 calories Men: 600 calories	Eats normally	Eats normally

Michael Mosley, a British journalist, popularized this diet, which is also known as the Fast Diet. On fasting days, women should consume 500 calories, and men should consume 600 calories. You might, for example, normally eat every day with the exception of Mondays as well as Thursdays. You eat two small meals of two hundred fifty calories each for women and three hundred calories each for men for those two days. You consume only five hundred to six hundred calories on two nonconsecutive days of the week using this method but normally eat on the other five days. All of these methods should help you lose weight by lowering your calorie intake, as long as you don't compensate by eating a lot more during the eating periods. The 5:2 diet is a simple intermittent fasting strategy. You normally eat five days a week and don't count calories. Then you cut your calorie intake to 1/4 of your daily requirements on the other two days of the week. For someone who consumes two thousand calories per day on a daily basis, this would entail cutting the calorie intake to 500 calories two days per week. According to a 2018 study, the 5:2 diet is almost as good for weight loss and blood glucose control in people with type 2 diabetes as daily calorie restriction. Another study found that the 5:2 diet was just as effective for weight loss as well as the mitigation of metabolic diseases such as heart disease and diabetes as continuous calorie restriction. The 5:2 diet allows you to choose which days you fast, and there are no restrictions on what or when you eat on full-calorie days. It's important to note that eating "normally" on full-calorie days does not imply that you can eat whatever you want. Even if it's only for two days a week, limiting yourself to five hundred calories per day is difficult. Furthermore, eating too few calories may cause you to become ill or faint. Although the 5:2 diet can be beneficial, it is not for everyone. Consult your physician to determine if the 5:2 diet is appropriate for you.

Eat Stop Eat

DAY 1	DAY 2	DAY 3	DAY 4	DAY 5	DAY 6	DAY 7
Eats normally	24-hour fast	Eats normally	Eats normally	24-hour fast	Eats normally	Eats normally

EAT-STOP-EAT

Once or twice a week, Eat Stop Eat involves a 24-hour fast. This amounts to a full 24-hour fast if you fast from dinner 1 day to dinner the next day. You've completed a full 24-hour fast if you successfully complete dinner at 7 p.m. Monday and don't eat again until dinner at 7 p.m. Tuesday. The end result is the same whether you fast from breakfast to breakfast or lunch to lunch.

During the fast, liquids such as coffee, water and other low-calorie beverages are permitted, but solid foods are not. It's critical that you eat healthily during the eating periods if you're trying to lose weight. In other words, you should eat as much as you would if you weren't fasting at all. Brad Pilon, author of the book "Eat Stop Eat," popularized an unconventional approach to intermittent fasting called "Eat Stop Eat." This intermittent fasting plan entails deciding on 1 or 2 non-consecutive days per week when you will go without eating for a 24-hour period. You can eat as much as you want the rest of the week, but it's best to eat a well-balanced diet and avoid overindulging. A weekly twenty-four hour fast is justified by the belief that eating fewer calories will result in weight loss. Fasting for up to twenty-four hours can cause a metabolic shift, causing your body to use fat instead of glucose as an energy source. However, abstaining from food for twenty-four hours at a time takes a lot of willpower and can lead to bingeing and overeating later. It could also result in disordered eating habits. To determine the Eat Stop Eat diet's health benefits as well as weight loss properties, more research is needed. Before you try Eat Stop Eat, talk to your doctor to see if it's a good weight-loss plan for you.

Alternate-day fasting

	ALTERNATE-DAY FASTING						
DAY 1	DAY 2	DAY 3	DAY 4	DAY 5	DAY 6	DAY 7
Eats normally	24-hour fast OR Eat only a few hundred calories	Eats normally	24-hour fast OR Eat only a few hundred calories	Eats normally	24-hour fast OR Eat only a few hundred calories	Eats normally

You fast on alternate days when you practice alternate-day fasting. This method was used in many of the test-tube studies that showed the beneficial effects of intermittent fasting. A complete fast every other day may seem excessive, so it is not advised for beginners. This method may cause you to go to bed hungry so many times per week, which is unpleasant and unlikely to be sustainable in the long run. Alternate-day fasting is a simple, easy-to-follow intermittent fasting plan. You fast every other day on this diet, but you could still eat anything you want on the non-fasting days. On fasting days, some versions of this diet follow a "modified" fasting method that includes eating around 500 calories. Other versions, on the other hand, completely eliminate calories on fasting days. Fasting on alternate days has been shown to help people lose weight. In a randomized pilot study of adults with obesity, alternate-day fasting was found to be equally good for weight loss as daily caloric restriction. Another study found that after alternating between 36 hours of fasting and 12 hours of unlimited eating for four weeks, participants consumed 35% fewer calories and lost an average of 7.7 pounds (3.5 kg). If you're serious about losing weight, incorporating an exercise routine into your daily routine can help. According to research, pairing alternate-day fasting with endurance exercise can result in weight loss that is twice as effective as simply fasting. Fasting for a full day every other day could be challenging, especially if you're new to the practice. On non-fasting days, it's easy to go overboard. If you're new to intermittent fasting, start with a modified fasting plan to ease into alternate-day fasting. It's important to remain a nutritious diet, utilizing high protein foods as well as low-calorie vegetables to help you feel full, whether you begin with a modified fasting plan or a full fast.

The Warrior diet

	DAY 1	DAY 2	DAY 3	DAY 4	DAY 5	DAY 6	DAY 7
Midnight							
4 AM	Eating only small amounts of vegetables and fruits	Eating only small amounts of vegetables and fruits	Eating only small amounts of vegetables and fruits	Eating only small amounts of vegetables and fruits	Eating only small amounts of vegetables and fruits	Eating only small amounts of vegetables and fruits	Eating only small amounts of vegetables and fruits
8 AM							
12 PM							
4 PM	Large meal	Large meal	Large meal	Large meal	Large meal	Large meal	Large meal
8 PM							
Midnight							

THE WARRIOR DIET

The Warrior Diet recommends eating small amounts of fruits and vegetables during the day and one large meal at night. The Warrior Diet is an intermittent fasting plan inspired by ancient warriors' eating habits. The Warrior Diet, developed by Ori Hofmekler in 2001, is more intense than that of the 16:8 method but also less restrictive than the Eat Fast Eat method. It entails eating very little during the day for 20 hours and then eating as much as desired during a four-hour window at night. During a 20-hour fast, the Warrior Diet motivates dieters to consume small amounts of dairy products, eggs that are hard-boiled, raw fruits & vegetables, and also fluids that have no-calorie. People can eat anything they want for a 4-hour window after a 20-hour fast, but healthy, unprocessed, and organic foods are recommended. While no research has been done on the Warrior Diet specifically, human studies have shown that time-restricted feeding cycles can help people lose weight. Other health benefits of time-restricted feeding cycles are unknown. In rodents, time-restricted feeding cycles have been shown to control diabetes, slow tumor growth, delay aging, and extend lifespan. More research on the Warrior Diet is needed to fully comprehend its weight-loss benefits. The Warrior Diet may be hard to adhere to because it limits calorie intake to only 4 hours per day. Overeating late at night is a common problem. The Warrior Diet has been linked to eating disorders. If you're up for the challenge, consult your physician to see if it's right for you.

1.5 Spontaneous meal skipping

	DAY 1	DAY 2	DAY 3	DAY 4	DAY 5	DAY 6	DAY 7
	Breakfast	Skipped Meal	Breakfast	Breakfast	Breakfast	Breakfast	Breakfast
	Lunch	Lunch	Lunch	Lunch	Lunch	Lunch	Lunch
	Dinner	Dinner	Dinner	Dinner	Skipped Meal	Dinner	Dinner

SPONTANEOUS MEAL SKIPPING

You don't have to stick to a strict intermittent fasting schedule to reap some of the benefits. Another option is to skip meals on occasion, such as when you aren't hungry or when you are too busy to cook and eat. It's a perception that women must eat every few hours or risk starvation or muscle loss. Your body is built to withstand long periods of hunger, let alone missing 1 or 2 meals every now and then. As a result, if you're not hungry 1 day, skip breakfast and eat a healthy lunch and dinner instead. Alternatively, if you're traveling and can't find anything to eat, go on a short fast. A spontaneous intermittent fast is when you skip 1 or 2meals when you feel like it. During the other meals, ensure to eat healthy foods.

1.6 The effects of Intermittent Fasting on Cells and Hormones

Quite a few things do happen in your body on a cellular and molecular level when you fast. To make stored body fat more accessible, your body adjusts hormone levels, for example. Essential repair processes and gene expression changes are also initiated by your cells. Although intermittent fasting can help with weight loss, it can also have a negative impact on your hormones. This is due to the fact that body fat is the body's method of securing energy (calories). When you don't eat, your body goes through a series of changes in order to make its stored energy more available. Adjustments in nervous system activity, as well as significant changes in the levels of several important hormones, are examples. Some of the changes that take place in the body when you fast are listed below:

Human Growth Hormone (HGH)

Growth hormone levels skyrocket, sometimes by as much as fivefold. This has a number of advantages, including fat loss and muscle gain.

Insulin

Insulin sensitivity improves, and insulin levels drop significantly. Insulin levels that are lower make stored body fat more available. When you eat, your insulin levels rise, and when you

fast, your insulin levels plummet. Insulin levels that are lower aid fat burning.

Cellular repair

When you fast, your cells begin to repair themselves. Autophagy is a process in which cells consume and remove the old and dysfunctional proteins which have accumulated inside them.

Gene expression

Improvements in the function of genes linked to longevity and disease resistance have been discovered.

Norepinephrine (noradrenaline)

Norepinephrine is a neurotransmitter that causes fat cells to break down body fat into free fatty acids, which can be burned for energy.

Bottom line

Interestingly, short-term fasting could increase fat burning, contrary to what some proponents of eating five to six meals per day claim. Alternate-day fasting trials of three to twelve weeks, along with whole-day fasting trials of 12–24 weeks, have been shown to reduce body weight and fat. Still, more research into the long-term effects of intermittent fasting is needed. Human growth hormone (HGH) is another hormone that changes during a fast, with levels rising up to five-fold. HGH was previously thought to aid fat burning, but new research suggests this could signal the brain to conserve energy, making weight loss more difficult. HGH may increase appetite and decrease energy metabolism by triggering a small population of agouti-related protein (AgRP) neurons. Fasting for a short period of time causes a number of physiological changes that aid fat loss. Nonetheless, rising HGH levels may have an indirect effect on energy metabolism, making it difficult to maintain weight loss. Intermittent fasting health benefits are due to hormonal changes, cell function, and gene expression.

1.7 Intermittent fasting is a very powerful weight-loss tool

The most popular reason for people to attempt intermittent fasting is to lose weight. Intermittent fasting can automatically reduce calorie intake by forcing you to eat fewer meals. Intermittent fasting also alters hormone levels, which aids weight loss. It increases the release of the fat-burning hormone norepinephrine in addition to lowering insulin as well as increasing growth hormone levels (noradrenaline). Short-term fasting could increase the metabolic rate by 3.6–14 percent as a result of these hormonal changes. Intermittent fasting leads to weight loss by altering both sides of the calorie equation by assisting you in eating fewer and burning more calories. Intermittent fasting has been shown in studies to be a very effective weight-loss tool. This eating pattern can result in 3–8% weight loss over 3–24 weeks, according to a 2014 review study, which is a significant amount when compared to most weight loss studies. People also lost 4–7% of the waist circumference, representing a high loss of harmful belly fat, which builds up around the organs and causes disease, according to the same study. In another study, intermittent fasting was found to cause less muscle loss than the more common method of constant calorie restriction. Keep in mind, however, that the main reason for its popularity is that intermittent fasting allows you to consume fewer calories overall. You may well not lose any weight if you binge and eat excessively during your eating periods. Intermittent fasting may help you eat fewer calories while slightly increasing your metabolism. It's a proven method for losing weight as well as belly fat.

Increase your fiber intake to improve your overall health and satiety between meals.

You should increase your intake of lean protein. If you want to increase your satiety and muscle mass, you'll need to do this. Individuals who successfully lost weight in a randomized controlled experiment of 12 months of alternate-day fasting reported increased protein intake, improved fullness, and reduced hunger when compared to those who did not lose weight, according to a study.

- You must stick to your calorie restrictions on fast days.
- On "feast" days, you should avoid high-energy meals and snacks.
- Early in the day, begin eating.

- Start eating within a specific time frame, especially on calorie-restricted days.
- You must eliminate added sugars from your diet.

1.8 Who should be careful or avoid it?

It's clear that intermittent fasting isn't for everyone. If you're underweight or even have a background in eating disorders, you must consult with a doctor before going on a fast. It can be outright dangerous in these situations.

1.9 Safety and Side Effects

The most common side effect of intermittent fasting is hunger. You may also feel tired, and your brain may not function as well as it once did. It may only be temporary, as your body will need time to adjust to the new meal schedule. Before attempting intermittent fasting, consult your doctor if you have a medical condition. This is especially crucial if you:

- Are you experiencing problems with blood sugar regulation
- Have low blood pressure
- Are Taking medications

- Have diabetes
- Are underweight
- Have a history of eating disorders
- Are you trying to conceive?
- Are you a woman and have a history of amenorrhea?
- Are breastfeeding or pregnant

1.10 Some popular questions and answers on Intermittent Fasting

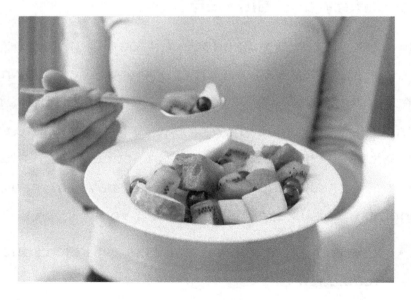

Here are answers to the most common questions about intermittent fasting.

Can one drink liquids during the fast?

Yes, you can drink non-caloric beverages besides water, coffee, and tea. Coffee should not be sweetened. It's possible that small amounts of milk or cream are acceptable. Coffee is especially beneficial during a fast because it suppresses hunger.

Is skipping breakfast unhealthy?

It is not true. The issue is that most stereotyped breakfast-skippers lead unhealthy lives. The practice is perfectly healthy if you ensure to eat healthy food for the rest of the day.

Can you take supplements during fasting?

Yes, supplements can be taken while fasting. Keep in mind, however, that some supplements, such as fat-soluble vitamins, may work better if taken with food.

Can you work out while you are fasting?

Fasted workouts are perfectly acceptable. Before a fasted workout, some people suggest taking branched-chain amino acids (BCAAs).

Does fasting result in muscle loss?

All weight loss methods could even result in muscle loss. That's why it's critical to lift weights and consume plenty of protein. Intermittent fasting tends to cause less muscle loss than regular calorie restriction, according to one study.

Does fasting slow down the metabolism?

There is no evidence to back it up. Short-term fasts have been shown in studies to boost metabolism. Fasting for three or more days, on the other hand, can slow down metabolism.

Can kids fast?

Your kids can fast under your supervision.

1.11 Intermittent fasting coupled with excellent ways to help lose weight after 50

Intermittent fasting is an eating pattern in which you only eat for a certain amount of time. The 16/8 method, in which you eat for 8 hours and then fast for 16, is the most common type of intermittent fasting. Intermittent fasting has been shown to help people lose weight in numerous studies. Furthermore, a few test-tube & animal studies may indicate intermittent fasting could benefit the old adults by extending the life, slowing the cell decline, as well as preventing age-related adjustments to mitochondria, your cells' energy-producing organelles. Though it may appear that weight loss becomes more difficult as you get older, there are many evidence-based strategies that can help you achieve as well as maintain healthy body weight after 50. Cutting added sugars from your diet, including strength training in your workouts, eating more protein, preparing meals at home, and eating a whole-foods-based diet are just a few of the ways to enhance your overall health as well as lose excess body fat. Maintaining a healthy weight as well as losing extra body fat could be hard for most adults as they are getting older. The gain of weight after the age of fifty may be caused by poor dietary choices, unhealthy habits, sedentary lifestyle & metabolic changes. However, regardless of the physical abilities or the medical diagnoses, at whatever age, you may lose weight by making few simple changes. The greatest ways to help you lose weight even after 50 are listed below.

You should enjoy strength training

Strength training's also important for women over 50, even though the cardio gets a great deal of attention once it arises to lose weight. Sarcopenia is a condition where muscle masses decline as you are getting older. Around 50 years of age, muscle mass loss begins, which may slow down metabolism & result in weight gain. So, after 50, the muscle mass declines at a rate of about 12% annually, while the muscle strength drops at a 1.5 to 5 % rate per year. As a result, including muscle-building workouts in your exercise routine is dangerous for preventing muscle loss related to age- & maintaining a healthy weight of the body. Strength training, like body-weight exercises, can improve muscle strength, size, & function significantly. Strength training may also help in losing weight by decreasing body fat & increasing the metabolism, which may help you burn more calories throughout the day.

Team up with a family member or friend

this may be hard to establish a healthy eating pattern as well as exercise the routine all upon your own. so, sticking to the plan as well as achieving the wellness goals may be easier only if you get together with a family member, coworker, or friend. According to the studies, those people who contribute to the weight-loss programs with the friends are much likely to maintain their weight less over time. Exercising with friends can also help in staying committed to the fitness program

& make this more enjoyable.

Burn calories by moving more

To lose the excess body fats, you should burn additional calories than consuming. That's why, when trying to lose weight, remaining more energetic throughout the day is critical. Sitting at the desk for a long period of time, e.g., may sabotage the efforts of weight loss. To combat it, simply moving up from the table & taking a 5-min walk each hour can help you to become far more active at work. So According to the studies, using Fitbit or a pedometer to track your steps can help you to lose weight by increasing activity & calorie expenditures. Start with a reasonable step aim based on the levels of current activity when using Fitbit or pedometer. Then, depending upon the overall health, slowly increase to seven thousand to ten thousand steps each day or even more.

Must increase your protein intake

It's critical to get sufficient protein of high quality in the diet for weight loss as it can also prevent or even reverse - muscle loss related to age. After 20 years of age, a number of the calories you might burn at rest, known as the resting metabolic rates (RMR), decreases by one to two % per decade. It's linked to muscle loss as people are getting older. A diet rich in protein-, on the other hand, may help prevent and even reverse muscle loss. Growing dietary proteins has also been shown in numerous studies to help in losing weight and keeping this off in the long run. Moreover, research demonstrates that older adults, particularly women over 50, have greater protein requirements than younger adults, stressing the significance of including foods that are protein-rich in the meals & snacks.

Talk to a dietitian

This may be hard to find an eating pattern that promotes weight loss while also nourishing your body. A registered dietitian may assist in determining the most effective method to lose extra fat without even having to follow a strict diet. Dietitian may also help to lose weight by giving support and guidance. Collaborating with a dietitian in losing weight can produce better consequences than going this alone, so according to the research, & it may also help maintain your loss of weight over time.

Try to cook and eat more at home

Several studies showed that the people who tend to

cook as

well as eat meals at their home have healthier diet & are not overweight than the ones who don't. When you're preparing meals at home, you've complete power over what might go into — & what remains out of — the recipes. This allows trying new, healthy ingredients which have piqued interest. Initiate by cooking 1 or 2 meals a week at the home if you consume most of your meals out. Then slowly increase the said number until you are cooking more at home than eating out.

Eat more vegetables and fruits

Vegetables & fruits are rich in nutrients which are vital for great health, & including them in the diet is a simple, scientifically proven method to lose weight. A review of 10 studies discovered which increasing daily veg servings was linked to 0.36 c.m or 0.14" waist reduction in the women. Another study found that eating fruits & vegetables reduced body weight, body fat & waist circumference in 26,341 men & women age 35 to 65.

Work with a personal trainer

So, working with a personal trainer may be especially beneficial for the ones who're new to exercise because they can teach you to workout properly to lose weight and avoid injury. The Personal trainers also could encourage you to work out more by making you responsible. They may even change the mind about exercising. A study of 10-week of 129 grown-ups found that one hour of 1-on-1 personal training per week increased exercise motivation & levels of physical activity.

Stay away from processed and convenience foods

now Eating convenience diets like candy, fast food & processed appetizers on a regular basis is linked to gaining weight & may sabotage your efforts of weight loss. Convenience food is rich in calories & low in some important nutrients like fiber, protein, vitamins & minerals. Fast food, along with different processed foods, is often mentioned as "the empty calories" for this reason. Scaling back on the convenience foods as well as substituting them with nutrient-rich whole food in nutritious meals & snacks is an intelligent way of losing weight.

Indulge in an activity which you love

It could be challenging for you to find an exercise routine that you may stick for a long period could be challenging. It is why it's critical to contribute to activities you enjoy. So, sign in for group sport as a running club or soccer, e.g., if you're enjoying group activities. This would allow to workout with others on a regular basis. So, if you choose solo activities, go for a solo ride or bike, solo walk, solo hiking, or solo swim.

Seek advice from a healthcare provider

If you're having trouble losing weight despite being active & eating a healthy diet, you should rule out conditions that can make it hard to lose weight, like hypothyroidism & polycystic ovarian syndromes (PCOS). It is particularly true if you've family members who suffer from the ailments. Tell the doctor about the symptoms so she or he can determine the best testing procedures to rule out any medical conditions that could be causing your weight loss problems.

Eat a diet that is based on whole foods

Sticking to a diet that is rich in full foods is 1 of the simplest ways to make sure that the body receives the nutrients it requires to thrive. Whole foods, like fruits, vegetables, nuts, poultry, seeds, legumes and fish, grains, are rich in protein, fiber, and healthy fats, which are important for maintaining a healthy weight of the body. Whole-foods-based diets, the plant-based & those that incorporate animal products, are linked to the loss of weight in numerous studies.

Do not eat excessively at night

Numerous studies show that consuming lesser calories at nighttime can help maintain a healthy weight & lose fat. Over the course of 6 years, the ones who consumed more calories at dinner were more than twice as likely to become obese as those who consumed more calories earlier in the day, according to a study of 1,245 people. Furthermore, those who consumed more calories at dinner were more likely to develop metabolic syndrome. It is a group of conditions that include high blood sugar and excess belly fat. Heart disease, stroke and diabetes are all increased by metabolic syndrome. Breakfast and lunch should contain the majority of your calories, with a lighter dinner being a viable option for weight loss.

Concentrate on your body composition

Although your body weight is an important indicator of health, your body composition, or the percentages of fat as well as fat-free mass in your body, is also important. Muscle mass, particularly in older women, is an important indicator of overall health. Your goal should be to gain more muscle while losing fat. There are several methods for calculating body fat percentage. Measuring the calves, waist, biceps, chest, and thighs, on the other hand, can help you figure out if you're losing fat as well as gaining muscle.

Keep yourself hydrated in a healthy manner

Drinks with added sugars and calories, such as soda, sweetened coffee beverages, sports drinks, juices and pre-made smoothies, are common. Sugar-sweetened beverages, particularly those sweetened with high-fructose corn syrup, have been linked to weight gain and diseases such as heart disease, obesity, diabetes and fatty liver disease. Substituting healthy drinks like water and herbal tea for sugary beverages can help you lose weight and lower the risk of developing the chronic conditions listed above.

Go for the right supplements

If you're tired and unmotivated, the best supplements can help you get the energy you would need to achieve your objectives. The ability to absorb certain nutrients decreases as you get older, increasing your risk of deficiency. Adults, particularly women over 50, are generally deficient in folate as well as vitamin B12, two nutrients required for energy production, according to research. B vitamin deficiencies, such as B12 deficiency, can affect your mood, induce fatigue as well as prevent you from losing weight. As a result, taking B-complex vitamins to help reduce the risk of deficiency is a good idea for women over 50.

Restrict added sugars

For weight loss at any age, limiting foods high in added sugar, such as ice cream, candy, sweetened beverages, cakes, cookies, sweetened yogurts and sugary cereals, is critical. Since sugar is added to so many foods, including things you wouldn't expect, such as salad dressing, tomato sauce and bread, reading the ingredient labels is the best way to find out if something has sugar added to it. Look for the words "added sugars" on the nutrition facts label, or look for common sweeteners like high-fructose corn syrup, cane sugar and agave in the ingredient list.

Look for ways for improving the sleep quality

The weight loss efforts may be damaged if you do not get sufficient good sleep. Sleep deprivations are linked to increasing the risk of obesity and have been shown to sabotage weight loss efforts in numerous studies. A two-year study of 245 women found that those who slept 7 hours or more per night were 33% more likely to lose weight than those who slept less than 7 hours per night. Weight loss success was also linked to better sleep quality. Reduce the amount of light in the bedroom and avoid using your phone as well as watching TV before bed to get the recommended seven to nine hours of sleep a night as well as improve your sleep quality.

Try to be more mindful

Mindful eating's a straightforward way to improve your relationship with the food while as well helping you to lose weight. Mindful eating involves paying closer consideration to whatever you eat and how you are eating. This helps you understand the hunger and fullness cues and also how food affects your mood & total well-being. Many of the studies have found that practicing mindful eating techniques helps people lose weight and improve their habits of eating. There aren't any hard & fast directions for heedful eating. However, eating slowly along with paying some attention to the color & taste of every bite and taking note of what you may feel during the meals are simple methods to start.

CHAPTER 2: Intermittent Fasting and its Health Benefits For Women Over 50

Intermittent fasting's a type of eating plan where you alternate between eating and fasting on a regular basis. Intermittent fasting showed in the studies to help people lose weight and prevent — or even reverse — disease. Many diets emphasize what to eat, but intermittent fasting emphasizes when to eat. Intermittent fasting is when you only eat at certain times of the day. Fasting for a set number of hours each day or eating only one meal a couple of times a week can aid in fat loss. Scientific evidence also suggests that there are some health benefits. Mark Mattson, Ph.D., a neuroscientist at Johns Hopkins University, has studied intermittent fasting for 25 years. He claims that our bodies have evolved to be able to go without food for several hours, days, or even weeks. Before humans learned to farm, they were hunters and gatherers who evolved to survive and thrive without eating for long periods of time. Hunting games and gathering nuts and berries took a lot of time and effort. It was easier to maintain a healthy weight even 50 years ago. Christie Williams, M.S., R.D.N., a dietitian at Johns Hopkins, explains. There were no computers available, and television shows ended at 11 p.m. Because they went to bed, people stopped eating. The portions were significantly smaller.

More people worked and played outside, getting more exercise in the process. Television, the internet, and other forms of entertainment are now available 24 hours a day, seven days a week. We stay up later to watch our favorite shows, play games and chat on the internet. We've grown accustomed to sitting and eating for most of the time of the day and night. Obesity, type 2 diabetes, heart disease, and other illnesses can all be exacerbated by consuming more calories and exercising too little. Intermittent fasting has been shown in scientific studies to help reverse these trends. Women can, on average, adopt a more flexible approach to fasting than men. Shorter fasting times, fewer fasting days, and/or eating a limited number of calories on fasting days are all possible choices.

2.1 Intermittent Fasting

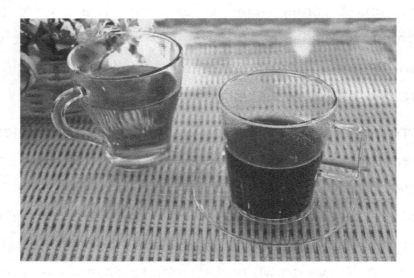

The world has been a victim of diet fads for a long. Diet pills were common in the 1990s. You were losing out on life's classic fitness boosts if you didn't own a juicer in the early 1980s. Green tea pads that minimize tummy size have been presented to us, and if you're not feeding like a Neanderthal, you're still at a disadvantage. Intermittent fasting is a common eating technique that is being researched in labs and used in kitchens all over the United States. And it isn't just a fad. Restricting the calorie intake or mealtimes can have a number of advantages, including weight loss and a lower chance of multiple diseases. Intermittent fasting limits whether and how much you eat — or both — for a period of time. There are a number of options.

Any second day, you regularly consume during alternate-day fasting. On the days in between, you consume just 25% of the daily calorie requirements in one meal. So, if you eat 1,800 calories on Monday, Wednesday, and Friday, then on Tuesday, Thursday, and Saturday, you'd eat a 450-calorie lunch (and nothing else). In the 5:2 diet, you eat regularly for five days and only consume only four hundred to five hundred calories for the next two days. Every day is the same for the 16:8 technique: you fast for 16 hours and only eat normally within eight hours, such as between 9 a.m. in the morning and 5 p.m. in the evening.

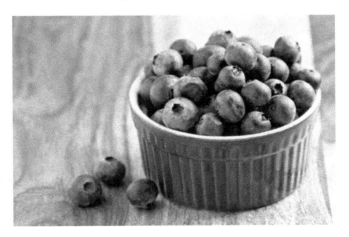

Intermittent fasting is a method of calorie restriction that involves a collection of on and off periods of consumption. It can seem to be a simple and straightforward task, but it is a test of self-control that can be frustrating initially. The first thing you'll find is that your belly fat is drastically reduced. Hormones also play a key role in fat reduction. Moreover, as we all know, weight gain in the midsection is a part of life during menopause.

2.2 The Technique

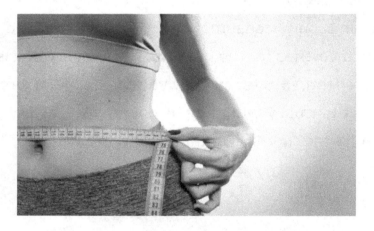

The act of reducing calories is a stimulus for weight reduction in and of itself, so it sounds like a no-brainer. A 12-hour fast is a perfect way to start your intermittent fasting journey. You'll have started your intermittent fasting experience once you finish your last meal before 8 p.m. and don't eat again until 8 a.m. the next day. The 12-hour fast will assist you in establishing a positive outlook and developing the consistency necessary to establish a regular eating schedule. When you've grown used to fasting for 12 hours, start experimenting with waiting until noon to eat your first meal. If you succeed, your body will have been abstaining for 16 hours. The next method is that you can fast for another four hours and then eat between 2 p.m. and 6 p.m. It is advised that you experiment to figure out what feels good to your body. You should never attempt a 20-hour fast without first preparing your body, but it is a challenge you should set for yourself if you want to shed more weight and feel fantastic. If you make it to midday, you've skipped one meal of the day, which means you've eaten 30% less (technically). Normally, weight loss is accomplished by eating less and exercising more, but animal experiments found that when mice overate outside of fasting hours, their longevity was only extended by 30%, suggesting that it is not so much what you consume but when you eat.

The science behind intermittent fasting

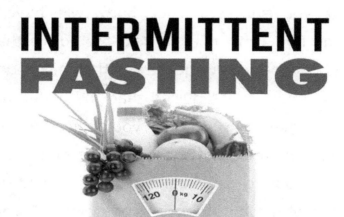

There's still some science at work here, in the form of your body's HGH production. Our bodies generate insulin to store glucose from carbohydrates so that it can be used later when we feel about eating something. We live in a world where most of our meals are routine, and we are constantly bombarded with foods that are rich in sugar and fat. This places us in an anabolic state, which means we're still adding weight. Food glucose is processed as fat, resulting in weight gain. Intermittent fasting effectively reverses this mechanism, allowing our cells to use the glucose that has been processed in our cells for energy. Weight loss occurs as cells reach a catabolic (breaking down) state. HGH is produced as a result of the body's need for glucose, but when we eat regularly, our HGH output is suppressed because we are receiving glucose from outside sources. HGH is a hormone that controls metabolism and has various advantages for muscle recovery and fat burning. HGH output can be increased by up to five times with intermittent fasting.

2.3 Best Intermittent Fasting Types for Women

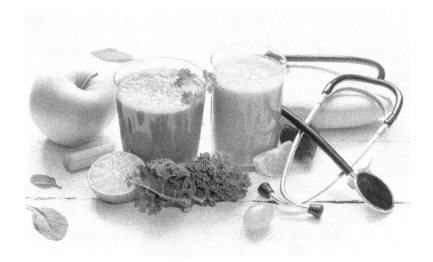

Given below are a few of the greatest types of intermittent fastings for women:

Crescendo Method

You could fast for 2 or 3 days a week for 12–16 hours. Fasting days should not be concurrent and should be spread out uniformly throughout the week (let us assume, Monday, Wednesday and Friday).

Eat-stop-eat (also called the 24-hour protocol)

Once or even twice a week, go on a complete 24-hr fast (it should not be practiced by more than two times a week for women). Begin with 14–16 hour fasts and work your way up.

The 5:2 Diet (also called "The Fast Diet")

The Fast diet works by restricting calories to 25% of your usual intake (about 500 calories). Moreover, you have to adhere to this style for two days a week and are allowed to eat "normally" for the remaining five days. You can have one day between fasting days.

Modified Alternate-Day Fasting

In this technique, you have to fast on alternate days. However, you are allowed to eat normally on non-fasting days. You are also permitted to consume 20–25% of your usual calorie intake (approximately 500 calories) on a fasting day.

The 16/8 Method (also called the "Lean gains method")

You are allowed to fast for 16 hours a day and consume all of your calories in an eight-hour cycle.

Women should begin with 14-hour fasts and work their way up to 16 hours. It is also necessary to eat well throughout the non-fasting hours, regardless of which option you chose. You do not enjoy the same weight loss and health effects if you consume a lot of fatty, calorie-rich foods during non-fasting times. It can easily be deduced from the said that the right solution is one that you can handle and maintain over time by not causing any negative health effects. Intermittent fasting can be done in a variety of forms by women. The 5:2 diet, modified alternate-day fasting and the crescendo method are three of the most effective approaches.

2.4 Getting started is quite easy

It's easy to get started. In reality, you've probably done a few intermittent fasts before. Often people eat this way out of habit, avoiding breakfast and dinner. The easiest way to getting started with intermittent fasting is to follow one of the intermittent fasting strategies mentioned above. You may not, though, have to adhere to a rigid timetable. Another choice is to fast anytime it is convenient for you. For certain people, skipping meals when they aren't hungry or don't have time to prepare the food may be beneficial. It doesn't matter the sort of fast you want at the end of the day. Finding a method that fits well for you and your lifestyle is the most critical thing.

2.5 Safety and Benefits of Intermittent Fasting

Many women feel safe by using modified forms of intermittent fasting. Hunger, low stamina, headaches, and poor breath are also possible side effects of intermittent fasting. Prior to beginning an intermittent fasting regimen, women who are pregnant, planning to conceive, or have a background of eating disorders must seek medical advice. Intermittent fasting is a dietary practice that includes short-term fasts on a daily basis. Regular 14–16-hour fasts, the 5:2 diet and/or modified alternate-day fasting is the safest for women. In both animals and humans, intermittent fasting has been suggested to influence the body and metabolism in a variety of ways. Fasting causes a "metabolic switch" from carb-burning to fat-burning, which is one of the most significant metabolic improvements.

Intermittent fasting for longevity

Another advantage of intermittent fasting is its anti-aging benefits and longevity value. This is largely done by autophagy, which is the body's normal means of removing weakened cells as well as replacing them with new, healthier ones. It's close to recycling. This is highly promising in terms of achieving long-term longevity. Intermittent fasting is a safe and effective way to replace old cells while also promoting the development of new ones. Autophagy is a natural phenomenon that our ancestors instilled in us to provide nutrition to the body (self-eating). Of course, this won't last forever, but because you'll be feeding all day, your body won't be able to sustain it. When our cells get stressed, intermittent fasting enhances autophagy. Autophagy is activated to protect and replenish the body. This literally prolongs our lives. According to studies, CR could extend the lifetime of rats by 30 percent. There are no medications or drugs involved, only a common trick that we can all use.

Intermittent fasting helps you reduce calories and lose weight

Intermittent fasting helps you eat fewer calories, which is why it helps you lose weight. During the fasting periods, all of the protocols require skipping meals. You will consume fewer calories except if you compensate through eating more during eating periods. Intermittent fasting helped reduce body weights by 3 to 8 % over a period of 3 to 24 weeks, according to a 2014 review. When it comes to weight loss, intermittent fasting has been shown to produce weight loss of 0.55 to 1.65 pounds (0.25–0.75 kilo gram) per week. The average waist of the participants reduced by four to seven inches. This indicated that they had lost belly fat. So, these findings suggest that intermittent fasting could be an effective weight-loss strategy. However, the advantages of intermittent fasting extend far beyond weight loss. Also, this has numerous metabolic health benefits and even may help lower the risk of heart disease. Although calorie counting's not necessary when doing intermittent fasting, loss of weight is primarily mediated by a reduction in overall calorie intake.

Intermittent fasting may help you maintain muscle mass

Dieting has the unfortunate side effect of causing muscle loss in addition to fat loss. Intermittent fasting has been shown in some studies to be beneficial in maintaining muscle mass while losing body fat. Intermittent calorie restriction resulted in similar amounts of loss of weight as continuous calorie restriction, yet with much smaller loss in the muscle mass, according to a scientific review. In calories restriction studies, muscle mass lost 25 % of weight lost, compared to 10percent in intermittent calories restriction studies.

Intermittent fasting makes healthy eating simpler

One of the main advantages of intermittent fasting for many people is simplicity. Most intermittent fasting plans only require you to keep track of time rather than calories. The best dietary pattern for you is one that you can maintain over time. If intermittent fasting is making it easier to follow a healthy diet, it'll have noticeable health & weight-loss benefits in the long run. Intermittent fasting has a number of advantages, one of which is that it makes healthy eating easier. In the long run, this may make it easier to hang to a healthy diet.

Weight Loss is quicker

Intermittent fasting, frequent or multi-day fasting and time-restricted eating have all been shown to aid weight control, boost metabolic health metrics, and lower the risk of cardiovascular disease and cancer, as augmented by various studies. Intermittent fasting's commonly done twice a week or every other day as a major or total energy restriction regimen.

Greater Insulin Sensitivity

Insulin sensitivity refers to how sensitive the body's tissues are to insulin's effects. Insulin sensitivity is affected by our level of physical exercise, sleep habits, the foods we consume, and also the time we eat. When compared with calorie restriction, alternate day fasting tends to be more effective at increasing insulin sensitivity and lowering fasting insulin. Another alternative to intermittent fasting's time-restricted feeding, which may target mechanisms and pathways linked to our circadian cycles, such as insulin sensitivity. Did you know that your metabolism varies during the day, depending on your internal biological clock, along with external influences like light sensitivity and food consumption? In the evening, for example, when your body is ready to burn fat as you sleep, you are usually more insulin tolerant (your tissues don't take up glucose as efficiently). In a study published in Cell Metabolism in 2018, Courtney Peterson and colleagues found that early time-restricted feeding, or eating during a 6-hour "feeding period" every day with breakfast about 8 a.m. and dinner before 3 p.m., increased blood pressure, insulin sensitivity, oxidative stress and appetite in men with pre-diabetes. And in the absence of weight loss, even certain health benefits were observed. What precisely does this imply? Metabolically, daily meal schedules that align food consumption with your circadian clock are beneficial. Metabolic health markers such as insulin sensitivity and low inflammatory factor levels are linked to a lower risk of heart disease, diabetes, and cancer.

Reduced Oxidative Stress and Inflammation

Oxidative stress happens as potentially damaging reactive oxygen species develop within metabolically active cells in the body. Reactive oxygen species (ROS) are reactive, as their name implies. Fasting on alternate days (or consuming every other day) has been shown to boost the expression of superoxide dismutase and catalase, two effective antioxidant enzymes that help the cells clean up reactive oxygen species (ROS). Exercising is another way to boost antioxidant enzymes. Physical exercise raises superoxide dismutase levels, which has many health effects for all of the body's organs.

Eat more fruits and vegetables

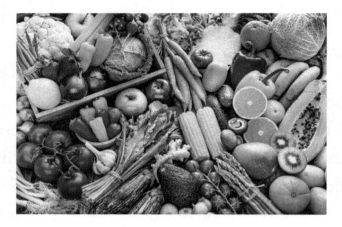

You need to increase your intake of plant-based green foods along with fruits and vegetables.

Exercise

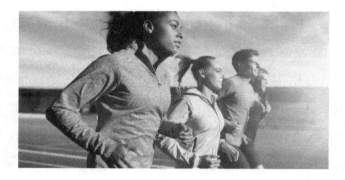

Though exercise is rarely a necessary activity for weight loss in and of itself, its health benefits extend well beyond weight loss. Physical activity and structured fitness will aid in weight management and the prevention of metabolic disorders like obesity and diabetes.

Maintain a balanced diet

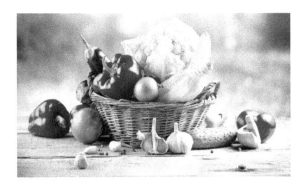

What you eat on a regular basis has an effect on your health along with how you feel in the present and future. Health plays a critical part in leading a healthier life. Your diet, when coupled with physical exercise, will help you achieve and sustain a healthier weight, lower your risk of chronic diseases like diabetes and heart disease, and improve your general health and well-being.

Avoid added sugars

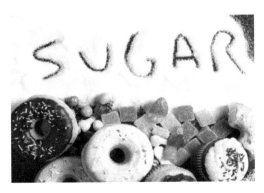

You must refrain from sugars and other simple

carbohydrates (white rice, white bread, etc.)

2.6 How to succeed with an intermittent fasting protocol

If you'd like to lose weight with intermittent fasting, there are a few things to keep in mind:

Food quality

It's still important to eat healthy foods. Eat whole or single-ingredient food as much as possible.

Calories

Calories are still important. During non-fasting periods, try to eat ordinarily, but not so many that you may compensate for calories you skipped while fasting.

Consistency

If you want it to work, you must stick with this for a long time, just like any other weight loss method.

Patience

It may take some time for your body to adjust to an intermittent fasting regimen. It will become easier if you are compliant with the meal schedule. Exercise, such as strength training, is recommended in almost all common intermittent fasting procedures. If you'd like to burn mainly body fats while keeping your muscle mass, this is crucial. When it comes to intermittent fasting, calorie counting's usually not necessary at first. Calorie counting, on the other hand, can be helpful if the weight loss plateaus. If you want to lose weight with intermittent fasting, you must still eat healthy as well as maintain a calorie deficit. Consistency is essential, as is regular exercise. Finally, intermittent fasting may be an effective weight-loss strategy. Its weight loss is primarily due to a reduction in calorie intake, but some of its hormone-related benefits may also play a role. Intermittent fasting may not be for everyone; however, it is extremely beneficial to women.

CHAPTER 3: A Guide For Women Over 50 On How To Start

Intermittent fasting allows you to eat fewer calories, lose weight, and reduce your diabetes & heart attack risks. Fasting, unlike other diets, doesn't really require calorie or macronutrient monitoring. In reality, there have been no dietary or dietary restrictions, making this more like a lifestyle than just a diet. Intermittent fasting's indeed a popular method to lose weight since it is an easy, quick and inexpensive way of eating less & lose body fat. It is also a growing aid in the prevention of diabetes and heart disease, the maintenance of muscle strength, and the improvement of mental well-being. Furthermore, since there are fewer meals to schedule, prepare, and serve, this eating style will help you conserve time at home. Intermittent fasting's a form of eating that involves periodic, brief fasts. It's just a common way of life that can help with the loss of weight, body composition, preventing disease, and overall well-being.

3.1 Intermittent fasting may affect men and women differently

Intermittent fasting might not be quite as effective for some females as it would be for males, according to some facts. In one research, women's blood glucose regulation deteriorated after 3 weeks of fasting, while men's glucose control improved. There were also several observational reports about women's menstrual periods changing since they began intermittent fasting. Since women's bodies are particularly vulnerable to calorie restriction, these changes arise. A small portion of the brain known as the hypothalamus is impaired when calorie consumption is limited, including when fasting for far too often or too long. Gonadotropin-releasing hormones (GnRH) is a hormone that aids in the activation of two sex hormones: luteinizing hormones (LH) & follicle-stimulating hormones (FSH). Whenever these hormones are unable to interact with the ovarian follicles, irregular cycles, miscarriage, poor bone strength, as well as other health problems may occur. While no equivalent human trials exist, 3 to 6 months with alternate-day abstinence in adult mice resulted in a decrease in uterus size and erratic menstrual cycles.

Women must take a changed solution to intermittent fasting, like shorter fasting times and fewer fasting days, both as a result of these factors.

3.2 Health benefits of intermittent fasting for women

Intermittent fasting will help you lose weight while still lowering the risk of contracting a variety of chronic diseases.

Heart Health

The main cause of death in the nation is cardiac arrest. Blood pressure, higher Cholesterol levels, and increased triglyceride levels are three of the most common risks for cardiac failure. Intermittent fasting reduced blood pressures by 6percent in only 8 weeks in a sample of 16 obese women and men. Intermittent fasting further reduced Cholesterol level by 25percent & triglyceride levels by 32 %, according to the same report.

Diabetes

Intermittent fasting will also enable you to treat your diabetes & lower your chances of contracting a disease. Intermittent fasting, including prolonged calorie restriction, tends to reduce certain diabetic risk factors. Mostly it accomplishes this by lowering the insulin levels & decreasing insulin tolerance. 6 months of intermittent fasting cut insulin level by 29percent and insulin tolerance by 19percent in a randomized controlled trial of even more than a Hundred overweight individuals. The amounts of blood sugar stayed unchanged. Furthermore, intermittent fasting for 8 to 12 weeks has also been found to decrease insulin levels by 20 to 31percent and blood glucose levels by 3 to 6percent in people with pre-diabetes, a disease wherein blood glucose levels are high but not severe enough just to diagnose diabetes.

Weight Loss

When performed correctly, intermittent fasting could be an easy and efficient way to reduce weight since brief fasts may help you eat less fat and lose weight. Several reports have found how intermittent fasting would be just as successful as a conventional calorie-restricted diet for losing weight in the short term. Intermittent fasting resulted in an overall weight reduction of 15 pounds (6.8 kilos) over the period of 3 to 12 months, as per a 2018 study of research in overweight individuals. Over a span of 3 to 24 weeks, intermittent fasting decreased body mass by 3 to 8percent in obese or overweight individuals, according to another study. Participants' waist measurements decreased by 3 to 7percent during the same time span, according to the report. Intermittent starvation seems to help with weight reduction in a brief period. The sum you lose, though, can most definitely be determined by how many calories you eat during the non-fasting hours and how well you stick towards the lifestyle.

It may help you eat less

Switching to intermittent fasting might help you eat less normally. When young male's food consumption was limited to four-hour duration, they consumed 650 lesser calories each day, according to one report. Another research looked at the impact of a lengthy, 36-hr fast to eating patterns of 24 active males and females. Despite eating more calories upon post-fast days, participants' overall calorie balance fell by 1900 kcal, a substantial decrease.

Reduced inflammation

Intermittent fasting has been shown in several trials to suppress essential inflammatory markers. Chronic inflammation may trigger weight gain & a slew of other health issues.

Improved psychological well-being

In one report, 8 weeks of intermittent fasting reduced stress & binge eating habits in obese adults, thus enhancing body appearance.

Cancer

Intermittent fasting has been shown in animal research to reduce the risk of cancer.

Brain health

Intermittent fasting boosts the brain hormones BDNF, which can help young nerve cells develop. It may even help to prevent Alzheimer's disease.

Anti-aging

Intermittent fasting has been shown to increase the lifetime of rats. The Fasted rats existed 36 to 83 percent longer, according to studies.

3.3 How does intermittent fasting work?

You won't have to deprive yourself when you practice intermittent fasting, also known as IF. Also, it doesn't owe you permission to eat a bunch of fatty food while you aren't fasting. Instead of consuming meals and treats during the day, you feed over a set period of time. A majority of citizens adhere to an IF regimen that allows everyone to fast for 12-16 hours per day. They enjoy regular meals and treats the majority of the day. Since most people are sleeping for around eight hours during their fasting times, sticking towards this feeding window isn't quite as difficult as it seems. You're often allowed to consume zero-calorie beverages like wine, tea, & coffee. You'll have the strongest effects from this plan if you stick to it. Around the same period, on rare days, you should certainly take a rest from this type of eating routine. You should try different types of intermittent fasting to see which one is well for you. Many people begin their IF journey with a 12 to 12 plan and then move to a 16-8 system. After that, continue to adhere to the schedule as closely as possible

3.4 What makes intermittent fasting work?

Some people claim that the IF has helped them lose weight mainly because the short eating window forces them to eat fewer calories. For example, instead of three meals and two snacks, they can only have space for two meals or one snack. People become more conscious about the foods they eat and prefer to avoid artificial carbohydrates, fatty fats, and simple carbs. Of course, you have the freedom to choose any nutritious foods you choose. While certain people use intermittent fasting to limit their daily calorie consumption, some use it in conjunction with keto, vegetarian, and other diets.

3.5 Is intermittent fasting healthy?

Remember how you can just fast for eight to twelve hours straight, not really for days. You also have plenty of time to eat a delicious and nutritious meal. Of course, certain older women could need regular eating due to metabolic diseases or drug guidelines. Under any scenario, you can talk to the doctor about your dietary patterns before implementing any adjustments. Although it isn't actually fasting, some physicians claim that enabling convenient foods like whole fruit, mostly during the fasting period, has health benefits. Adjustments like this will also provide a much-needed break for the digestive & metabolic systems. For, e.g., the famous weight-loss textbook "Fit for the Life" recommended consuming just fruit after supper but before lunch. In reality, according to the writers of this novel, they had clients who just modified their eating patterns by fasting for 12-16 hours per day. Despite not adhering to diet's other guidelines or counting calories, they shed weight and improved their fitness. This technique may have failed largely because dieters swapped fast food with whole food. In either scenario, participants considered this dietary modification to be beneficial and simple to implement. Traditionalists won't name this fasting, so it's good to remember that you do have choices if you cannot go without eating for more than a few hours.

3.6 Is intermittent fasting the best technique?

In medical literature, there are few drawbacks of the IF. It's how the blood sugar and insulin levels can plummet throughout the fasting phase. The body will depend on accumulated fat for energy if insulin's hormone fat-storing mechanism is not present. In either scenario, IF seems to succeed, which is why it's relatively simple to follow. By reducing consumption windows, it lets you automatically reduce calories & make healthier food decisions. According to some research, IF tends to encourage fat loss whilst sparing muscle mass, making it a safer option than just reducing calories, fat, or carbs. Many studies have been done on intermittent fasting in both animals and humans. These studies have shown that it can have **powerful benefits** for weight control and the health of your body and brain. It may even help you **live longer**.

3.7 You can lead a care-free life

Good eating is easy, but this can be difficult to sustain. One of the most significant barriers is the amount of time and effort taken to schedule and prepare nutritious meals. Intermittent fasting will make life simpler, so you don't have to prepare, serve, or tidy up quite so many meals as you would otherwise. Intermittent fasting's also very common among the life-hacking community, as it increases your wellbeing while also simplifying life.

3.8 Tips to keep an intermittent fasting diet on track

Intermittent fasting is gaining popularity, and with it comes concerns about how to bring the best out of the weight-loss technique. The advantages are obvious, the programs are simple to execute, and most do not need calorie counting. Intermittent fasting has been shown to improve people's wellbeing and can also prolong the onset of Alzheimer's disease symptoms. Intermittent fasting doesn't really cause eating problems or cause people's metabolism to hold back. The very first five quick days are challenging, but once your body adjusts to the up-and-down eating routine, it becomes quite easy. The strategies mentioned below will help you increase your odds of succeeding with intermittent fasting.

Consult your doctor

Before beginning the diet, always consult the doctor. Patients with Type One, diabetes breastfeeding mothers, & lactating women should avoid intermittent fasting. It form of regimen would not fit those with eating disorders, so they will appear to overeat through their diet plan.

Give due consideration to the intermittent fasting plan during the selection process

The 16:8 method, also known as time-restricted eating, involves fasting for sixteen hours per day and eating whatever you like for the remaining eight hours. Since your body's less effective at storing sugar as the day progresses, experts recommend choosing an eating time that allows you to complete your meals reasonably early, like Ten a.m. to 6:00 p.m. or sooner. Alternate days fasting entails restricting the calories by 500 calories a day, and consuming anything you like next, and so forth. The 5:2 diet entails integrating two different short days into the week, followed by regular eating on the remaining days.

Ways to suppress hunger during intermittent fasting

Following techniques can help you take control of your hunger during intermittent fasting.

Eat high-fiber foods

You should eat. During your feeding window, consume high-fiber items like almonds, beans, vegetables and fruits, as well as protein-rich foods like beef, seafood, nuts, or tofu. High-fiber gummies may also be beneficial.

Drink lots of water

People also mistakenly believe they are starving while they are actually thirsty; as a result, when intermittent fasting, individuals must drink plenty of fluids.

Black coffee, tea, cinnamon or licorice herbal teas are recommended drinks

The beverages might have an appetite-suppressing effect.

Watch less TV

This might seem odd, but then you are often bombarded by food advertisements when viewing television. This will leave you feeling hungry when you're not even really hungry. Remember that just being hungry is really the greatest thing that might happen to anyone. It creates a real mind-body bond that aids in recognition of fullness.

When should you exercise?

A study was conducted that Fasting but also exercises on alternating days. The volunteers in the research were given the option of exercising on fasting or feasting day, but there is no clear choice for one reason or another. However, researchers were shocked to learn that dieters felt more energized on the fasting days. So, in just this case, exercise before eating because individuals get starving about 30 minutes after finishing their workout and may find it difficult to keep to their diet if they cannot consume food afterward.

Workout before or after the 16:8 feeding window if you're following the 16:8 diet. Saving food after your gym session, whether you're performing alternating day fasting & running on the 500-calories day.

Skipping breakfast

The idea that missing breakfast is terrible for the waistline probably came from experiments funded by cereal producers, and the majority of the study focused on the impact of skipping breakfast on children's memory. Breakfast isn't the most effective meal for losing weight, according to a 2015 report. Obesity and diet studies found no statistical evidence to suggest a correlation between consuming breakfast & losing weight or missing breakfast and gaining weight in another study.

Ways to combat feelings of low energy and low focus

You can follow the following techniques to help you counter feelings of low energy.

Try drinking black coffee

this helps **in improving concentration & energy** but doesn't have any calories in it.

Take a deep breath and give yourself a break

A little meditation and mindfulness will go a far toward making you feel comfortable during your fasting time.

3.9 The best foods to eat on an Intermittent Fasting diet

Water & zero-calorie drinks, including black coffee & tea, are allowed on days that you aren't consuming. And "regularly eating" during your cycles does not imply "going insane." If you fill your meals with high-calorie fast food, extremely fried foods, &desserts, you're not going to drop weight or be healthy. Intermittent fasting, on the other hand, helps you to consume and appreciate a variety of foods. Having to eat with others and enjoying the mealtime moment, in general, increases happiness and promotes good health. Please consult a health practitioner before making any major dietary changes to ensure that it is the right choice for you. Intermittent fasting is creating quite a buzz in the overpopulated world of diet and exercise, including the word's sinister connotation. A substantial amount of evidence, though with small sample sizes, shows that diet will result in weight loss and better blood glucose levels. It's no surprise that everybody and the aunt have jumped on the IF bandwagon. Perhaps the attraction stems from the absence of food regulations. There are limitations to where and when you should consume, but not always on what you can buy. What portion, however, is also crucial. In between the fasts, you shouldn't be eating pints of frozen yogurt and packets of popcorn, which is why we've compiled a collection of the best things to eat on an IF diet.

Best foods and drinks you should be using when you are on intermittent fasting

There are no specifications or restrictions about what type or how much food to eat while following intermittent fasting. However, the advantages of intermittent fasting are unlikely to be accompanied by a steady diet of Burgers. Losing weight, retaining energy levels, & keeping to a diet both require a very well diet. Nutritional foods such as fruits, vegetables, whole grains, almonds, beans, dairy, seeds & lean proteins can be prioritized for those trying to lose weight. If you consume enough of the foods mentioned below, you will not get hungry when fasting.

3.10 Best drinks for intermittent fasting

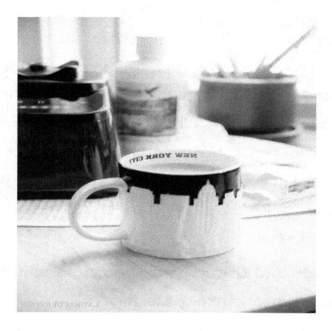

Fasting in between meals is a good way to increase stamina, improve mental focus, and lose weight. While not eating is an integral part of that too, what you consume between those is equally important. Here, I'm going to tell you about the right foods and drinks to eat while doing intermittent fasting. Fasting's a situation where one goes without eating for a period of time. It's not a novel concept.

Fasting has indeed been practiced for centuries for social and cultural reasons, although there has lately been a renewed emphasis on fasting regarding health reasons.

This not only helps you lose weight but that also strengthens your mental clarity, allows you more stamina, lowers your blood pressure, and extends your life.

During fast, you can avoid eating but not consuming. In reality, liquids are essential for staying hydrated. You should also consume those drinks when fasting to enjoy all of the advantages. The below are top picks:

Water

Water is a no-brainer. Steady sipping on H2O will keep you hydrated while fasting. This isn't actually a snack, but it's crucial for making it through the IF. the Water is important for the protection of almost all of the body's main organs. Avoiding this is a component of the quick will be stupid. Your organs play a critical role in your survival. The volume of water that each individual can drink depends on their gender, weight, height, level of exercise, and environment. However, the color of urine is a strong indicator. For all occasions, you want that to be yellow in color. Dehydration, which may induce headaches, nausea, and light-headedness, is shown by deep yellow urine. When you combine that with a lack of calories, you have a formula for catastrophe or, at very least, very darkened pee. If warm water doesn't appeal to you, try adding a splash of lemon juice, several mint leaves, or the cucumberslices to all of it. And here is why H2O reigns supreme.

Bone broth

In contrast to regular broth or bone, the broth is high in nutrients, including calcium, magnesium, & some other minerals, and also collagen, a protein that is necessary for healthy skin, joints, & hair. Bone broth's a form of liquid fuel which has been shown to enhance joint health & replenish electrolytes, all of which are essential during a swift.

Bone broth (or vegetable broth) is recommended for any time you decide to fast for 24 hours or more. While it has calories, it does not contain any carbohydrates, so it helps you stay in ketosis.

Black Coffee

Black coffee has no calories and has no impact on insulin levels. Through fasting windows, we should drink daily (caffeinated) and decaf coffee; really, don't add extra sweetener or cream. Coffee may help with hunger suppression during fast, and it must be served without sugar or milk. And sure, you don't consume more than 50 calories in a day. Cinnamon and other spices are perfectly appropriate. During fasting periods, many coffee lovers indulge in a cup of coffee, or even espresso, without any negative consequences. However, if you consume coffee throughout the fasting window, so you can feel a pounding heart or a disturbed stomach, so keep an eye on your own encounter. Black coffee can help to enhance a few of the advantages of intermittent fasting, but it's a common choice among keto dieters. Caffeine appears to help with ketone development, according to a report. Coffee has been found to help maintain stable blood glucose levels over time.

Herbal teas

Herbal teas provide the same benefits as do water. The Tea with no caffeine is a perfect way to keep hydrated and will also help you lose weight. If you're fasting, make sure you drink it without milk or sugar. With the tea, you will naturally improve the satiety. It may be the hidden tool that makes the fasting strategy not just simpler and more effective. Color, orange, oolong, & herbal teas are all suitable for consumption during a short. Tea helps to make intermittent fasting more successful by promoting gut wellbeing, probiotic balance, & cellular health. The Green teas, in fact, have been shown to aid in weight loss by increasing satiety.

Benefits of green tea (Pique Tea)

Fasting and green tea were used for health purposes for centuries, and they complement each other beautifully. Green tea reduces hunger, thereby rising fat burning, & fasting stimulates the protective curing state of autophagy. The Green tea abstinence removes body fat, strengthens the intestine and recharges the microbiota, and reduces inflammation in such a synergistic way. To have green tea whilst also fasting is a great way to increase both of these effects. The leaves & leaf bud of the Camellia sinensis, a tiny leafy tree native of East Asia, are used to make green tea. Color, orange, white, yellow, oolong, & fermented teas are all made from tea leaves that have been handled differently. Green tea's produced from the tea leaves, which haven't been through as much oxidation as black tea has because caffeine content is lower as well as the polyphenol content is higher. Polyphenols being plant products with a wide range of health advantages. There are hundreds of common polyphenols. Catechins seem to be the most common polyphenols throughout tea, with epigallocatechin gallate is now the most abundant (EGCG). Herbal tea leaves often contain other protective flavonoids, including quercetin. Antioxidants within green tea, such as EGCG, may be anti-inflammatory, & depending on use, green tea may have a variety of health benefits.

Green Tea Health Benefits

- Green tea may help with wrinkles
- Green tea may help with weight loss
- Green tea may help improve blood pressure
- the Green tea's beneficial to the eyes.
- Green tea will help to keep blood sugar levels in check.
- Green tea may help lower cholesterol levels in the blood.

Using high-quality green tea like the Pique Tea as green tea's fasting since it is safe from oxidation & pollution, and the cold brewing method they use raises the volume of green tea antioxidants by up to 12 times. Pique teas have a biochemical impact after just 2 to 3 cups, while a medicinal dosage of green tea needs 10 to 12 cups. This creates a huge change when doing green tea early so the hunger-suppressing and the fat-burning impact of green tea would be stronger.

Apple Cider Vinegar

ACV appears to aid in the maintenance of normal blood sugar levels & digestion. It could also help the intermittent fasting schedule work better. If you don't like the taste of AVC, try this as a dressing of salad at mealtimes. It's beneficial at every time during the day.

Benefits of Bulletproof Coffee for Women

Though black coffee is allowed throughout IF, Bulletproof Coffee's a common way of breaking the quick. It's blended with good-quality chocolate, grass-fed oil, & MCT oils for just a brain-boosting drink that's both high in calories and good fats. Mornings may be tough. Like most people, You actually don't function very well until you've had your first pot of joe. Things settle down afterward, and the planet becomes a happier environment. For you, as you will discover when you will read, the only thing greater than just a good cup of coffee in the morning is a decent cup of coffee in the afternoon.

What is Bulletproof Coffee?

You will experience many positive benefits when you start drinking bulletproof coffee. Above all, it is also very delicious. Essentially, it's made with freshly-roasted, high-quality beans, grass-fed butter, & MCT, or the Brain Octane Oils. Caprylic lipids are focused in MCT & Brain Octane. The MCT is Nine times more powerful than coconut oil, which also contains these important fatty acids, & Brain Octane's Eighteen times stronger. You can also add butter to bulletproof coffee. Butter should not cause weight gain. Our bodies do not really know where to go with toxic artificial fats, not a little amount of vitamin K-rich grass-fed oil. It's a question of perspective; however, a morning bagel or muffin with butter and jelly likely has much more butter, unlike your coffee. Once the butter is melted into the coffee, it makes it the most delectable, smooth, rich texture and flavor you'll ever taste. It also tends to hold you feeling full for hours & suppresses your appetite. The following are some of the benefits of using grass-fed butters:

- Omega-3 fats, beta-carotene, CLA, vitamin A,

vitamin KD, vitamin K, vitamin E, & antioxidants are all stronger in butter (grass-fed) than in grain-fed butters. The disparity of appearance between grass-fed and grain-fed or factory-farmed butters is visible: grass-fed butters are a bright yellow, whereas grain-fed or factory-farmed butters are almost white. The absence of color indicates that butter was generated by weakened, nutrient-depleted cattle.

- Butyrate, short-chained fatty acid, was abundant in the grass-fed butters. Butyrate has been shown in clinical studies to both inhibit and reduce inflammation. Butyrate has been shown to defend against mental disease, enhance body structure, boost metabolism, & improve intestinal health in rodents in experiments.

You can also add oil to the coffee

You do not have to add cheap cooking oils to your coffee. You can add MCT Oil or (Brain Octane Oils) is a combined source of the healthy essential fats contained in the coconut oil. While molten coconut oil has several advantages. Caffeine, found naturally in the coffee, aids in the transfer of medium-chained triglycerides across the blood-brain barrier, bypassing the liver altogether and thereby providing the brain with the vital nutrients it requires. MCT oil is also known as brain octane oil. It is Antibacterial & anti-inflammatory effects are found in acids fatty acids. Coconut oil contains it, but the Brain Octane oil's 18 times stronger.

The benefits of drinking bulletproof coffee

Given below are the benefits of drinking bulletproof coffee:

- Long-lasting stamina gain
- Little post-caffeine collapse
- Ability to concentrate on constructive tasks for hours
- Reduce sugar cravings, which are most certainly the result of energy dumps.
- No further coffee withdrawal symptoms or headaches
- You'll be ready to concentrate for four hours at a time.

When you will do Intermittent Fasting, you will find that Bulletproof coffee's the only way you would like to break your fast.

Recipe for classic bulletproof coffee

Ingredients

Given below are the ingredients that will be used for making a delicious cup of bulletproof coffee.

- Eight to twelve ounces of Upgraded Coffee (brewed)
- One tbsp MCT Oil or Brain Octane
- One tbsp unsalted grass-fed, ghee or butter

Instructions

Given below are the step-by-step instructions that you should follow for making a delicious cup of bulletproof coffee.

- Brew one cup (eight to twelve ounces) of the coffee in a coffee brewer (French press) or the pour-over method with filtered water.
- Fill a blender halfway with brewed coffee. 1 tablespoon MCT oil or Brain Octane and one tbsp grass-fed butters in a blender
- Blend for twenty to thirty seconds or until coffee froths up like latte foam. Pour into a mug of your choice and enjoy.

3.11 The drinks that you must avoid during intermittent fasting

You can be surprised to learn that several drinks (such as "zero-calorie" drinks) may help you split your high. This implies that consuming these can cause the body to wake up from its quick. On your quick, we'll discuss details regarding popular drinks like diet drinks, coconut water, almond milk, and alcohol.

You must avoid drinking a diet soda while intermittent fasting.

About the fact that diet soda has no calories, it's uncertain how sugar substitutes can affect fasting.

Can you use almond milk and coconut water while intermittent fasting?

Almond milk & coconut water also have a lot of sugar in them. Since sugar equals carbohydrates, you will be no longer deemed to have been fasting until you drink them. You should stop consuming these at the times that you are fasting.

And what about using alcohol while intermittent fasting?

It's safer to keep alcohol intake to your feeding periods

on days when you are intermittent fasting. Since most alcoholic drinks are full of sugar & calories, breaking the fast with alcohol is simple. Furthermore, alcohol has a stronger effect on an empty stomach, but just one bottle of wine consumed within a fasting period might make you feel worse the very next day.

Best foods to break an intermittent fast

Though BulletProof Coffee would be a perfect way to end the fast, you can also try consuming several foods to help you break the Intermittent Fasting time. To get the most out of IF, make sure you get the majority of your calories from the nutrient-dense products during your "eating" windows. Selecting whole meals to make healthy meals can keep you energized and help the body absorb nutrients more effectively during fasts. The Lean proteins must be consumed to split the quick. Chicken, pork, beef, turkey, fish, & eggs are among the better proteins for breaking a short. You can also eat healthier fats to crack the fast. Bulletproof, as previously said, seeds, grass-fed butter, almonds, avocados, nut butters, coconut oil, olive oil, and coffee are all great ways to split the fast with good fats. When on intermittent fasting, we can make this a priority to consume as many vegetables as you choose.

Consume one helping of fruit as well. A portion of berries, whether raw or frozen, is a tasty way to get micronutrients. This will assist you with keeping the blood sugar level in check. Because of concentrated quantities of the sugars per meal, canned fruits and juice should be avoided. Complex carbohydrates could also be included. Sweet potatoes, beans, quinoa, white potatoes, barley, and other full grains are often used and are extremely filling. To crack your hard, you can ideally avoid the high foods and instead concentrate on healthier protein and fat. To put it another way, miss cereal and go for fried eggs or omelet instead. Given below is the breakdown of recommended foods and their benefits.

Avocado

Eating the greatest fruit when attempting to lose some weight can appear counterintuitive. The Avocados, on the other hand, can hold you complete through even the shortest fasting times thanks to the high unsaturated fats content. Unsaturated fat, according to research, helps hold the body healthy even though you do not feel hungry. Your body sends out signals that it doesn't need to be in emergency hunger mode because it's enough calories. And if you're starving in the midst of fasting time, unsaturated fats hold these symptoms running much longer. Another research showed that using half avocado with your lunch will help you stay full for longer hours than that if you don't consume green, mushy fruit.

Fish and seafood

There's an explanation why American Dietary Recommendations recommend 2 or 3 4-ounce portions of fish each week. In contrast to being high in good fats and proteins, it is also high in vitamin D. But if you like to feed at short window times, do you not want to get more nutritious bang for the buck while you do? You will not run short of options to prepare fish since there are too many options.

Cruciferous veggies

Fiber is abundant in foods such as cabbage, Brussels sprouts, & cauliflower. It's important to consume fiber-rich foods at frequent intervals to hold you regularly & ensure that the poop factory goes smoothly. Fiber will also help you feel whole, which is beneficial if you won't be able to feed for another 16 hrs. Cruciferous vegetables can also help you avoid cancer.

Potatoes

It is important to note that not all white food is bad. Potatoes are found to be among the most nourishing foods in 1990s research. In addition, a 2012 study showed that using potatoes in a balanced diet can aid weight loss.

Beans and legumes

On IF diet, your favorite chili topping might be the best pal. Food, especially carbohydrates, provides energy for physical exercise. It isn't a good idea to carbohydrate-load to insane proportions, but including low-calorie carbohydrates like beans & legumes in the diet can't hurt. This will help you stay awake through your fasting period. Furthermore, ingredients like black beans, chickpeas, peas, & lentils have indeed been proven to help people lose weight, particularly though they aren't on a diet.

Probiotics

Consistency and variety appeal to critters in the stomach. If they're starving, this means they're not comfortable. And if your stomach isn't comfortable, you may notice any unpleasant side effects, such as constipation. Add probiotic-rich products like kombucha, sauerkraut and kefir to the diet to combat this unpleasantness.

Berries

These smoothie classics are packed with vitamins and minerals. That isn't even the most exciting aspect. People who ate a lot of flavonoids, like those used in strawberries and blueberries, had lower BMI rises over a 14-year span than people who didn't even eat berries, according to a 2016 report.

Eggs

One big egg has 6.24 grams of protein & takes just minutes to prepare. And, particularly when you are eating less, having quite enough protein as necessary is critical for staying full as well as building muscle. Males who had eggs breakfast rather than a bagel have been less hungry & ate less during the day, according to a 2010 survey. To put it another way, if you are searching for something else to do throughout your quick, why not boil those eggs? And, when time is perfect, you should consume them.

Nuts

Nuts have more calories than most other chips, but they often have healthy fats, which are lacking in most snack foods. Even don't be concerned with calories. According to a 2012 report, a 1-ounce portion of almonds (roughly 23 nuts) contains 20% fewer calories than label claims. Chewing does not fully break down cell walls of almonds, according to the report, which keeps a part of the nut safe and prevents it from being absorbed by the body through digestion. As a result, eating almonds may not cause as much of a difference in your regular calorie consumption as you would think.

Whole grains

Dieting and carbohydrate use tend to fall under two distinct categories. That's not always the case, as you will be glad to learn. Since whole grains are high in fibre and nutrition, a small amount would keep you satisfied for a long time. So, get out of the comfort zone & try farro, spelled, bulgur, Kamut, millet, amaranth, freekeh, or sorghum, whole-grain fantasy land.

3.12 Intermittent fasting side effects

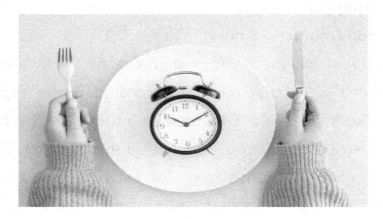

Intermittent fasting has grown in popularity over the last few years due to its promises of enhanced health and weight loss.

The idea is that cutting calories drastically a few times a week or limiting eating to a shorter "eating window" each day is easier than cutting calories moderately at every meal, every day. Extending fasting periods improve insulin sensitivity, enhance cellular repair, increase levels of human growth hormone, improve insulin sensitivity as well as change gene expression in a way that encourages longevity and disease prevention, according to proponents. However, there are some dangers. Because there are several types of intermittent fasting, some plans may trigger more side effects than others, but it's important to talk to a doctor about the following intermittent fasting side effects before deciding on a plan that fits your lifestyle.

Intermittent fasting may make you feel sick

Individuals may experience lethargy, headaches, crankiness and constipation depending on how long they fast. You may also want to switch from ADF fasting to periodic fasting or even a time-restricted eating framework that helps you to eat every day within a certain time period to reduce some of these unwanted side effects.

It may cause you to overeat

Since the appetite hormones, as well as hunger center in the brain, go into overdrive when you are deprived of food, there is a strong biological push to overeat after fasting periods. Because it's human nature to want to reward ourselves after putting in a lot of effort, such as exercising or fasting for a long time, there's a risk of indulging in unhealthy eating habits on non-fasting days. Two common side effects of calorie-restricted diets—slowed metabolism and increased appetite—are just as probable when people practice intermittent fasting as when they reduce calories every day, according to a 2018 study. And the evidence is mounting in studies of time-restricted eating that is out of sync with a person's circadian rhythm.

It may be dangerous if you're taking certain medications

If you want to try intermittent fasting, make sure you talk to your doctor first. For people with certain illnesses, such as diabetes, skipping meals as well as drastically reducing calories can be dangerous. Some people who take blood pressure or heart disease medications may be more susceptible to sodium, potassium, and other mineral imbalances during longer-than-normal fasting periods. Fasting may be difficult for people who really need to

3.13 Why does intermittent fasting result in constipation in some people?

The Changes in the diet can easily result in bowel movement changes. People who fast intermittently may experience constipation as a result of dehydration & lack of dietary fiber. If you are eating lesser now as the window-eating's limited, it is possible you're not getting sufficient nutrients, particularly dietary fiber, to keep the bowel movements steady. Dietary fiber aids the proper functioning of the digestive system by bulking up the stool and ensuring that food passes easily through the digestive tract. As a result, not getting sufficient of this can lead to a low number of toilet visits. The same is true if you don't drink enough water or other fluids. Fiber is only effective if you get enough fluids in your diet, so if you do not drink enough water, it can make this even more difficult for the stool to cross. If you're following an extreme method of intermittent fasting, such as the OMAD diet, you're probably drinking a lot less water. The lesser water you drink, the more likely you are to become constipated. The lesser water you consume during a fast, the longer it lasts. It's also important to remember that the foods contain water. Constipation is defined as having lesser than 3 bowel movements per week or going three days without a bowel movement. However, you may still

have constipation and pass stool. Constipation is defined by large, hard, dry stools that require draining to pass.

3.14 What if you're having the problem of diarrhea?

Even though you might believe that your new diet is to accuse of the looser stools, this may not be the case. Diarrhea is rarely caused by fasting alone. However, there are a variety of causes of diarrhea. Lactose intolerance or certain medications are the most common and harmless causes. So, 1 plausible explanation that you have added something latest to the diet that you didn't realize you were allergic to, such as dairy products. Or else, consider if there are any other underlying causes for your diarrhea, such as new medication, irritable bowel syndromes, celiac disease, thyroid disorder, or a colon infection, among others.

3.15 Keep your bowel movements regular while you are on intermittent fasting

Constipation can be avoided by eating additional fibre as well as drinking additional water, mostly during the non-fasting time of intermittent fasting.

Up your fibre intake

Active individuals should consume 25-30g of fibre in a day.

Getting sufficient fibre in your diet will help to ensure that the stool is thick to pass & that it does so smoothly. There are numerous foods rich in fibre that you can include in your diet, ranging from sweet potatoes to Brussels sprouts.

Drink enough water

3 to 4 liters of water per day is the recommended daily intake. Helping the stool to move along requires a combination of water and fibre.

Drink coffee

Coffee may make you want to go to the bathroom as soon as 4 minutes after you drink it. The mechanism of the action, believe it or not, is still a mystery. What we actually do know's that coffee causes receptors in colons to contract, & caffeine is not thought to be the cause.

Get active

Bowel motility is stimulated by physical activity. A sedentary lifestyle, on the other hand, could be a factor contributing to constipation. Increased bowel motility reduces the time stool spends in the colon, which reduces the amount of the water absorbed from the stool, making it less dry, hard, and difficult to pass.

Furthermore, any exercise will stimulate bowel motility, though aerobic exercise may be the most effective because it improves the flow of blood to all the organs, such as the gastrointestinal tract.

Conclusion

Intermittent fasting has become a popular health trend in recent years. It's said to help people lose weight, improve their metabolic health, and possibly even live longer. This eating pattern can be approached in a variety of ways. Every method has the potential to be effective, but determining which one works best for you is a personal decision. Intermittent fasting can be done in a variety of ways. It is also an accepted fact that reduced metabolism, achy muscles along with sleep problems and reduced muscle mass make it more difficult to lose weight after 50. Simultaneously, losing fat, including dangerous belly fat, will significantly lower the risk of major health problems, including heart attacks, diabetes and cancer. Of course, when you get older, the chances of contracting a variety of diseases increase. When it comes to weight loss and reducing the risk of contracting age-related diseases, intermittent fasting for women over fifty can become a virtual fountain of youth in some cases. You won't have to starve yourself if you practice intermittent fasting, also known as IF. It also doesn't give you permission to eat a variety of fatty food when you aren't fasting. Rather than consuming meals and snacks during the day, you eat over a set period of time. The majority of people stick to an IF plan that allows them to fast for twelve to sixteen hours a day. They enjoy regular meals and snacks the majority of the day. Since most people sleep for around eight hours during their fasting hours, sticking to this eating style isn't as difficult as it seems. You're also allowed to drink zero-calorie beverages like tea, coffee and water. For optimal intermittent fasting outcomes, build an eating routine that fits you. For example, if you're on a 12-12 fast, then you could miss breakfast and eat at lunch. You might eat an early supper and skip evening snacks if you want to eat your morning lunch. A 12-12 fast is relatively easy to maintain for older women. A 16-8 IF plan can help you achieve faster results. Within an 8-hour span, most people prefer to eat two meals and a snack or two. For instance, the eating window may be fixed between noon and 8 p.m., or between 8 a.m. and 4 p.m., However restricted meal times may not be suitable for you on a daily basis. Another choice is to follow a twelve or sixteen-hour fast for five days and then rest for two days. For example, you might do intermittent fasting throughout the week and eat regularly on the weekends. On alternating days, another variation calls for severely calorie-restricted eating. For instance, you might restrict your calories to less than 500 calories on one day and then eat the next day sensibly. It's worth noting that regular IF fasts never necessitate calorie restrictions that low. You'll have the best results from this diet if you stick to it. Around the same time, on rare days, you should certainly take a break from this kind of eating routine. You should try various forms of intermittent fasting to see which one is best for you. Many people begin their IF journey with the 12-12 plan and then move to the 16-8 plan. After that, continue to adhere to the schedule as closely as possible. People assume that IF has helped them lose weight because the short eating window naturally makes them consume fewer calories. For example, instead of three meals and two snacks, they can only have time for two meals and one snack. They become more aware of the foods they eat and prefer to resist refined sugars, harmful fats and empty calories. Of course, you have the freedom to eat whatever nutritious foods you choose. While some people use intermittent fasting to limit their daily calorie consumption, some use it in conjunction with a keto, vegan, or other diets. Although some nutritionists believe that IF only succeeds because it encourages people to eat less, others argue. They assume that with the same number of calories and other nutrients, intermittent fasting produces greater effects than traditional meal schedules. Studies have also proposed that fasting for several hours a day accomplishes more than mere calorie restriction. These are some of the metabolic modifications that IF induces, which can help explain the synergistic effects. Lower insulin levels during the fasting cycle can aid fat burning. HGH levels increase as insulin levels fall, promoting fat burning and muscle development. The nervous system will deliver this chemical to cells in reaction to an empty stomach, informing them that they must release fat for fuel. Intermittent fasting is a healthy way to eat. Know that you can only last for 12 to 16 hours at a time, not for days. You also have plenty of time to eat a delicious and nutritious meal. Of course, certain older women may require regular feeding due to metabolic diseases or drug instructions. In any case, you can speak to the doctor about your dietary habits before making any adjustments. Although it isn't actually fasting, some physicians claim that allowing easy-to-digest foods like whole fruit during the fasting window has health benefits. Modifications like this will also offer a much-needed break for the digestive and metabolic processes. IF seems to succeed mostly because it is relatively simple to follow. By reducing eating windows, it makes people automatically reduce calories and make healthier food decisions. If you've had trouble losing weight because your diet didn't fit or was too difficult to adhere to, you need to try intermittent fasting for the most effective and desired results.

CPSIA information can be obtained
at www.ICGtesting.com
Printed in the USA
BVHW061131170621
609531BV00013B/1275